PLANT-BASED SJOGREN SYNDROME DIET FOR SENIORS

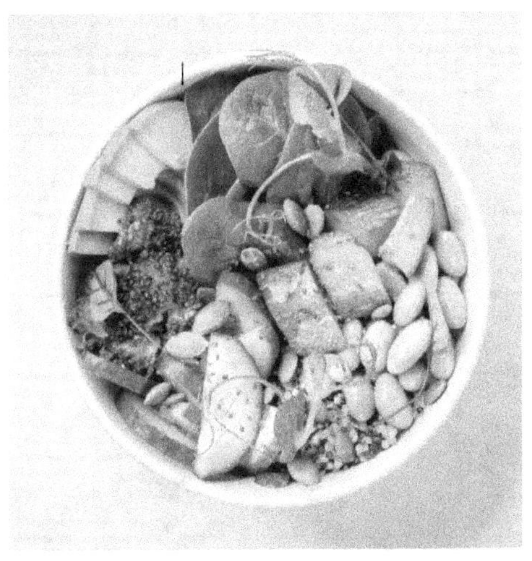

DR. JESSICA SMITH

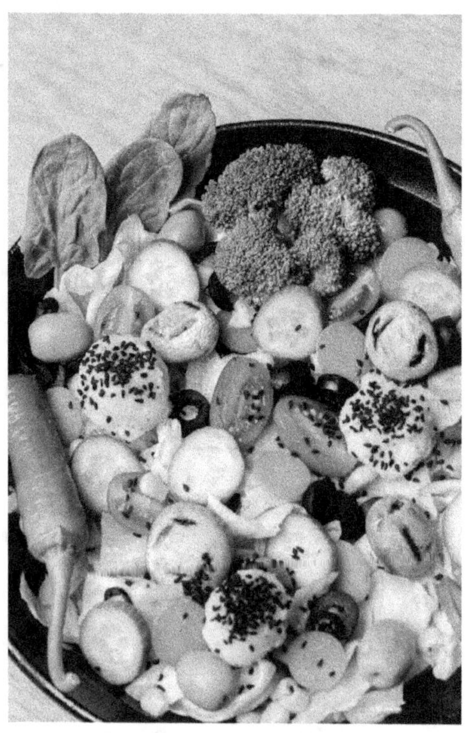

TABLE OF CONTENTS

CHAPTER ONE

How to Use this Cookbook

Consult with a healthcare provider: Before making any significant dietary changes, it's important for seniors with Sjögren's syndrome to consult with their healthcare provider or a registered dietitian who can provide personalized recommendations based on their health status and individual needs.

Focus on whole plant foods: Emphasize consuming a variety of whole plant foods such as fruits, vegetables, whole grains, legumes, nuts, and seeds. These foods are rich in vitamins, minerals, antioxidants, and fiber which can help support overall health and alleviate symptoms associated with Sjögren's syndrome.

Stay hydrated: Sjögren's syndrome can cause dry mouth and eyes, so it's essential for seniors to stay well-hydrated. Encourage consuming plenty of water throughout the day and incorporating hydrating foods such as cucumbers, watermelon, and soups into meals.

Incorporate omega-3 fatty acids: Omega-3 fatty acids have anti-inflammatory properties that may help reduce inflammation associated with Sjögren's syndrome. Include plant-based sources of omega-3s such as flaxseeds, chia seeds, walnuts, and hemp seeds into the diet regularly.

Limit processed foods: Minimize the consumption of processed and refined foods such as sugary snacks, desserts, processed meats, and fried foods. These foods can contribute to inflammation and may exacerbate symptoms of Sjögren's syndrome.

Experiment with herbs and spices: Herbs and spices not only add flavor to meals but also offer various health benefits. Incorporate herbs and spices like turmeric, ginger, garlic, and cinnamon into cooking to help reduce inflammation and enhance immune function.

Include probiotic-rich foods: Probiotics can promote gut health and support the immune system. Incorporate fermented foods such as sauerkraut, kimchi, tempeh, and non-dairy yogurt into the diet to introduce beneficial bacteria to the gut.

Opt for healthy fats: Choose sources of healthy fats such as avocados, olives, nuts, and seeds to support heart health and reduce inflammation. These fats can also help improve the absorption of fat-soluble vitamins from plant foods.

Mindful eating: Encourage seniors to practice mindful eating by paying attention to hunger and fullness cues, chewing food slowly, and savoring each bite. This approach can help improve digestion and nutrient absorption.

Be flexible and enjoy variety: A plant-based diet offers a wide range of delicious and nutritious foods to explore. Encourage seniors to experiment with new recipes, ingredients, and cuisines to keep meals interesting and enjoyable while meeting their nutritional needs.

Understanding Plant-Based Sjogren Syndrome Diet for Seniors

Understanding the nuances of a plant-based diet tailored for seniors with Sjögren's syndrome involves a multifaceted approach that integrates nutritional science, symptom management, and individual preferences.

Sjögren's syndrome, an autoimmune condition characterized by dry eyes and mouth, among other symptoms, necessitates dietary considerations to alleviate discomfort and support overall health.

A plant-based diet emphasizes whole, minimally processed foods derived from plants, such as fruits, vegetables, whole grains, legumes, nuts, and seeds.

For seniors with Sjögren's syndrome, focusing on hydration is paramount due to the propensity for dry mouth and eyes. Incorporating water-rich foods like cucumbers and watermelon, along with adequate fluid intake, helps maintain hydration levels.

Furthermore, emphasizing omega-3 fatty acids from plant sources like flaxseeds and walnuts can help mitigate inflammation associated with the condition.

However, individualized approaches are crucial, considering seniors' unique nutritional requirements and any coexisting health conditions. Consulting healthcare providers or registered dietitians can ensure that seniors with Sjögren's syndrome receive personalized dietary recommendations tailored to their needs, optimizing their overall health and quality of life.

Principles of Plant-Based Sjogren Syndrome Diet for Seniors

The principles of a plant-based diet for seniors with Sjögren's syndrome revolve around maximizing nutrient intake to manage symptoms and promote overall health. Here are some key principles:

Whole Foods Emphasis: Prioritize whole, unprocessed plant foods such as fruits, vegetables, whole grains, legumes, nuts, and seeds.

These foods provide essential nutrients, fiber, and antioxidants that support immune function and reduce inflammation, which is particularly important for seniors with Sjögren's syndrome.

Hydration: Since Sjögren's syndrome often leads to dry mouth and eyes, staying hydrated is crucial. Encourage seniors to consume plenty of fluids, including water and hydrating foods like soups, fruits, and vegetables.

Omega-3 Fatty Acids: Include plant-based sources of omega-3 fatty acids such as flaxseeds, chia seeds, walnuts, and hemp seeds. Omega-3s have anti-inflammatory properties that may help alleviate symptoms associated with Sjögren's syndrome.

Probiotics: Incorporate probiotic-rich foods like fermented vegetables, tempeh, and non-dairy yogurt into the diet to support gut health and enhance immune function.

Antioxidants and Anti-inflammatory Foods: Focus on foods rich in antioxidants and anti-inflammatory compounds, such as berries, leafy greens, turmeric, ginger, and garlic, to help reduce inflammation and oxidative stress.

Balanced Nutrition: Ensure a balanced intake of macronutrients (carbohydrates, protein, and fats) and micronutrients (vitamins and minerals) to support overall health and well-being.

Individualized Approach: Tailor the plant-based diet to meet the individual needs and preferences of seniors with Sjögren's syndrome, considering factors such as food tolerances, medication interactions, and personal dietary goals.

It's essential for seniors to work closely with healthcare providers or registered dietitians to develop a personalized plant-based diet plan that meets their specific needs and goals.

Benefits of Plant-Based Sjogren Syndrome Diet for Seniors

A plant-based diet tailored for seniors with Sjögren's syndrome offers numerous benefits that can significantly impact their overall health and well-being:

Reduced Inflammation: Plant-based diets are rich in anti-inflammatory compounds such as antioxidants, phytonutrients, and omega-3 fatty acids. By reducing inflammation, seniors may experience decreased pain and discomfort associated with Sjögren's syndrome.

Improved Hydration: Many plant-based foods, such as fruits and vegetables, have high water content, aiding in hydration for seniors experiencing dry mouth and eyes due to Sjögren's syndrome.

Heart Health: Plant-based diets are naturally low in saturated fats and cholesterol, promoting heart health and reducing the risk of cardiovascular diseases, which may be elevated in individuals with autoimmune conditions like Sjögren's syndrome.

Weight Management: Plant-based diets tend to be lower in calories and higher in fiber compared to omnivorous diets, making them beneficial for weight management. Maintaining a healthy weight can help alleviate stress on the body and reduce inflammation.

Gut Health: The fiber-rich nature of plant-based diets promotes a healthy gut microbiome, which is essential for immune function and overall health. Probiotic-rich foods commonly found in plant-based diets further support gut health and may enhance immune system modulation.

Nutrient Density: Plant-based diets are rich in vitamins, minerals, and phytonutrients, providing seniors with essential nutrients to support immune function, bone health, cognitive function, and overall vitality.

Digestive Health: The high fiber content of plant-based diets can promote regular bowel movements and alleviate constipation, a common issue for seniors with Sjögren's syndrome.

However, it's essential for them to work with healthcare professionals to ensure their dietary choices meet their individual nutritional requirements and health goals.

Tips for Plant-Based Sjogren Syndrome Diet for Seniors

Transitioning to a plant-based diet for seniors with Sjögren's syndrome can be made easier with the following tips:

Start Gradually: Begin by incorporating more plant-based meals into the senior's diet gradually. This allows for adjustment and exploration of new foods without overwhelming them.

Focus on Variety: Encourage seniors to experiment with a wide variety of plant foods to ensure they receive a diverse range of nutrients. Include fruits, vegetables, whole grains, legumes, nuts, seeds, and plant-based proteins in their meals.

Meal Planning: Help seniors plan their meals ahead of time to ensure they have nutritious plant-based options readily available. This can prevent reliance on convenience foods and make meal preparation easier.

Educate on Substitutions: Teach seniors about plant-based alternatives to their favorite animal-based foods. For example, they can use tofu or tempeh instead of meat, and plant-based milk alternatives like almond or soy milk instead of cow's milk.

Hydration: Remind seniors to stay hydrated by drinking water throughout the day and consuming hydrating foods like fruits and vegetables.

Cooking Methods: Encourage seniors to explore different cooking methods such as steaming, baking, roasting, and stir-frying to enhance the flavor and texture of plant-based foods.

Snack Smart: Provide healthy plant-based snack options such as fresh fruit, nuts, seeds, or veggie sticks with hummus to curb hunger between meals.

Supplementation: Discuss with healthcare providers or dietitians if supplementation with nutrients like vitamin B12, vitamin D, or omega-3 fatty acids is necessary to ensure seniors meet their nutritional needs on a plant-based diet.

Community Support: Connect seniors with support groups, online forums, or cooking classes focused on plant-based eating to provide encouragement, inspiration, and practical tips from others following similar dietary patterns.

Listen to Preferences: Respect seniors' food preferences and tastes while encouraging them to explore new plant-based foods and flavors at their own pace.

Guidelines for Plant-Based Sjogren Syndrome Diet for Seniors

Guidelines for a plant-based diet tailored to seniors with Sjögren's syndrome provide a structured approach to optimize nutrition and manage symptoms.

Here are some essential guidelines:

Consult Healthcare Providers: Before making significant dietary changes, seniors should consult with healthcare providers or registered dietitians to ensure the diet meets their nutritional needs and complements their treatment plan.

Focus on Whole, Minimally Processed Foods: Emphasize consuming a variety of whole plant foods, including fruits, vegetables, whole grains, legumes, nuts, and seeds, to maximize nutrient intake and minimize inflammation.

Stay Hydrated: Due to the prevalence of dry mouth and eyes in Sjögren's syndrome, seniors should prioritize hydration by drinking water regularly and consuming hydrating foods like fruits, vegetables, and soups.

Omega-3 Fatty Acids: Incorporate plant-based sources of omega-3 fatty acids such as flaxseeds, chia seeds, walnuts, and hemp seeds to help reduce inflammation and support heart health.

Antioxidants and Anti-inflammatory Foods: Include foods rich in antioxidants and anti-inflammatory compounds, such as berries, leafy greens, turmeric, ginger, and garlic, to help manage inflammation and oxidative stress associated with Sjögren's syndrome.

Probiotics: Incorporate probiotic-rich foods like fermented vegetables, tempeh, and non-dairy yogurt to support gut health and enhance immune function.

Monitor Nutrient Intake: Seniors should monitor their intake of essential nutrients such as protein, calcium, vitamin D, vitamin B12, and iron to ensure they meet their nutritional needs on a plant-based diet.

CHAPTER TWO

1. Overnight Chia Seed Pudding

Ingredients:

> - 1/4 cup chia seeds
> - 1 cup non-dairy milk (such as almond or coconut milk)
> - 1 tablespoon maple syrup or honey (optional)
> - Fresh fruits for topping (e.g., berries, sliced banana)

Instructions:

> - In a bowl, mix chia seeds, non-dairy milk, and sweetener (if using). Stir well.
> - Cover and refrigerate overnight or for at least 4 hours.
> - In the morning, stir the pudding and top with fresh fruits.
> - Serve chilled.

Health Benefits:

- ➤ Chia seeds are rich in omega-3 fatty acids, fiber, and antioxidants, which can help reduce inflammation and promote heart health.
- ➤ This breakfast is hydrating and provides essential nutrients.

Preparation Time: 5 minutes (plus chilling time)

2. Berry and Spinach Smoothie

Ingredients:

- ➤ 1 cup fresh spinach
- ➤ 1/2 cup mixed berries (e.g., strawberries, blueberries, raspberries)
- ➤ 1 ripe banana
- ➤ 1 cup non-dairy milk (e.g., almond milk)
- ➤ 1 tablespoon chia seeds (optional)
- ➤ Ice cubes (optional)

Instructions:

- ➤ Place all ingredients in a blender.
- ➤ Blend until smooth and creamy.

> Add more non-dairy milk if needed to reach desired consistency.

> Pour into glasses and serve immediately.

Health Benefits:

> This smoothie is packed with vitamins, minerals, antioxidants, and fiber from the spinach and berries, supporting immune function and reducing inflammation.

> Chia seeds add omega-3 fatty acids for heart health.

Preparation Time: 5 minutes

3. Avocado Toast

Ingredients:

> 1 ripe avocado

> 2 slices whole grain bread

> Cherry tomatoes, sliced (optional)

> Sprouts or microgreens (optional)

> Lemon juice (optional)

> Salt and pepper to taste

Instructions:

> Toast the bread slices until golden brown.

- ➢ Mash the avocado in a bowl and season with lemon juice, salt, and pepper.
- ➢ Spread the mashed avocado evenly onto the toasted bread slices.
- ➢ Top with sliced cherry tomatoes and sprouts or microgreens, if desired.
- ➢ Serve immediately.

Health Benefits:

- ➢ Avocado provides healthy fats, vitamins, and minerals, while whole grain bread adds fiber for digestive health.
- ➢ This breakfast is hydrating and nutrient-dense.

Preparation Time: 10 minutes

4. Oatmeal with Almond Butter and Berries

Ingredients:

- ➢ 1/2 cup rolled oats
- ➢ 1 cup water or non-dairy milk
- ➢ 1 tablespoon almond butter
- ➢ Mixed berries (e.g., strawberries, blueberries, raspberries)

- ➢ Maple syrup or honey (optional)
- ➢ Chopped nuts or seeds (optional)

Instructions:

- ➢ In a saucepan, bring water or non-dairy milk to a boil.
- ➢ Stir in the rolled oats and reduce heat to low. Cook for 5-7 minutes, stirring occasionally, until thickened.
- ➢ Remove from heat and stir in almond butter until well combined.
- ➢ Transfer oatmeal to a bowl and top with mixed berries, maple syrup or honey, and chopped nuts or seeds, if desired.
- ➢ Serve warm.

Health Benefits:

- ➢ Oats are rich in fiber, which aids digestion and helps stabilize blood sugar levels.
- ➢ Almond butter provides healthy fats and protein, while berries offer antioxidants and vitamins.

Preparation Time: 10 minutes

5. Tofu Scramble

Ingredients:

- 1/2 block firm tofu, crumbled
- 1/4 cup diced bell peppers
- 1/4 cup diced onions
- Handful of spinach
- 1/2 teaspoon turmeric powder
- Salt and pepper to taste
- 1 teaspoon nutritional yeast (optional)
- Cooking oil

Instructions:

- Heat a skillet over medium heat and add cooking oil.
- Add diced bell peppers and onions to the skillet and sauté until softened.
- Add crumbled tofu to the skillet and sprinkle with turmeric powder, salt, pepper, and nutritional yeast (if using). Stir well to combine.
- Cook for 5-7 minutes, stirring occasionally, until tofu is heated through and lightly browned.
- Add spinach to the skillet and cook for an additional 2-3 minutes until wilted.

> Remove from heat and serve hot.

Health Benefits:

> Tofu is a good source of plant-based protein and calcium, while bell peppers and spinach provide vitamins and antioxidants.

> Turmeric has anti-inflammatory properties.

Preparation Time: 15 minutes

6. Quinoa Breakfast Bowl

Ingredients:

> 1/2 cup cooked quinoa

> Sliced banana

> Chopped nuts (e.g., almonds, walnuts)

> Dried fruit (e.g., raisins, cranberries)

> Cinnamon

> Maple syrup or honey (optional)

Instructions:

> In a bowl, layer cooked quinoa, sliced banana, chopped nuts, and dried fruit.

> Sprinkle with cinnamon and drizzle with maple syrup or honey, if desired.

➢ Serve warm or cold.

Health Benefits:

➢ Quinoa is a complete protein, providing all essential amino acids, and is rich in fiber and minerals.
➢ Bananas add potassium and natural sweetness, while nuts offer healthy fats and protein.

Preparation Time: 10 minutes (if quinoa is pre-cooked)

7. Sweet Potato Breakfast Hash

Ingredients:

➢ 1 medium sweet potato, diced
➢ 1/2 bell pepper, diced
➢ 1/2 onion, diced
➢ Handful of kale or spinach, chopped
➢ 1 teaspoon smoked paprika
➢ Salt and pepper to taste
➢ Cooking oil

Instructions:

➢ Heat a skillet over medium heat and add cooking oil.

- ➢ Add diced sweet potato to the skillet and cook for 5-7 minutes, stirring occasionally, until slightly softened.
- ➢ Add diced bell pepper and onion to the skillet and continue cooking for another 5 minutes until vegetables are tender.
- ➢ Stir in chopped kale or spinach, smoked paprika, salt, and pepper. Cook for an additional 2-3 minutes until greens are wilted.
- ➢ Remove from heat and serve hot.

Health Benefits:

- ➢ Sweet potatoes are rich in vitamins A and C, fiber, and antioxidants.
- ➢ Bell peppers and leafy greens add more vitamins and minerals, while smoked paprika adds flavor without added salt.

Preparation Time: 20 minutes

8. Banana Pancakes

Ingredients:

- ➢ 1 ripe banana

- ➤ 1/2 cup rolled oats
- ➤ 1/4 cup non-dairy milk
- ➤ 1/2 teaspoon baking powder
- ➤ 1/2 teaspoon vanilla extract
- ➤ Maple syrup or fruit for topping (optional)

Instructions:

- ➤ In a blender, combine banana, rolled oats, non-dairy milk, baking powder, and vanilla extract. Blend until smooth.
- ➤ Heat a non-stick skillet over medium heat and lightly grease with cooking oil.
- ➤ Pour pancake batter onto the skillet to form pancakes of desired size.
- ➤ Cook for 2-3 minutes on each side until golden brown.
- ➤ Serve warm with maple syrup or fresh fruit toppings, if desired.

Health Benefits:

- ➤ These pancakes are gluten-free and naturally sweetened with banana, making them suitable for various dietary needs.

> ➤ Rolled oats provide fiber and slow-releasing energy.

Preparation Time: 15 minutes

9. Coconut Yogurt Parfait

Ingredients:

> ➤ 1 cup coconut yogurt (or any non-dairy yogurt)
> ➤ 1/4 cup granola
> ➤ Mixed berries
> ➤ Coconut flakes (optional)
> ➤ Maple syrup or honey (optional)

Instructions:

> ➤ In a glass or bowl, layer coconut yogurt, granola, and mixed berries.
> ➤ Repeat layers until ingredients are used up.
> ➤ Sprinkle with coconut flakes and drizzle with maple syrup or honey, if desired.
> ➤ Serve immediately.

Health Benefits:

> ➤ Coconut yogurt is a dairy-free alternative rich in probiotics, which support gut health and immune function.

> ➢ Granola adds crunch and fiber, while berries provide antioxidants and vitamins.

Preparation Time: 5 minutes

10. Veggie Breakfast Burrito

Ingredients:

- ➢ Whole grain tortilla wraps
- ➢ Scrambled tofu (see recipe #5)
- ➢ Sliced avocado
- ➢ Sautéed bell peppers and onions
- ➢ Fresh salsa or pico de gallo
- ➢ Fresh cilantro (optional)
- ➢ Lime wedges (optional)

Instructions:

- ➢ Heat tortilla wraps in a skillet or microwave until warm and pliable.
- ➢ Fill each tortilla with scrambled tofu, sliced avocado, sautéed bell peppers and onions, fresh salsa, and cilantro, if desired.
- ➢ Roll up the tortilla to form a burrito.
- ➢ Serve with lime wedges on the side for squeezing.

Health Benefits:

> ➢ This breakfast burrito is packed with plant-based protein, healthy fats, and fiber, providing sustained energy and essential nutrients. It's a satisfying and flavorful way to start the day.

Preparation Time: 20 minutes (if preparing scrambled tofu)

Plant-Based Sjogren Syndrome Diet Lunch Recipes for Seniors

1. Quinoa Salad with Chickpeas and Lemon-Tahini Dressing

Ingredients:

> ➢ 1 cup cooked quinoa
> ➢ 1/2 cup cooked chickpeas (canned is fine)
> ➢ Mixed greens (e.g., spinach, arugula)
> ➢ Cherry tomatoes, halved
> ➢ Cucumber, diced
> ➢ Red onion, thinly sliced
> ➢ Lemon-Tahini Dressing: 2 tablespoons tahini, 2 tablespoons lemon juice, 1 tablespoon water, 1 clove garlic (minced), salt and pepper to taste

Instructions:

> ➤ In a large bowl, combine cooked quinoa, chickpeas, mixed greens, cherry tomatoes, cucumber, and red onion.
> ➤ In a separate small bowl, whisk together tahini, lemon juice, water, minced garlic, salt, and pepper to make the dressing.
> ➤ Pour the dressing over the salad and toss to coat evenly.
> ➤ Serve immediately or refrigerate until ready to eat.

Health Benefits:

> ➤ Quinoa and chickpeas provide protein and fiber, while vegetables offer vitamins, minerals, and antioxidants. The lemon-tahini dressing adds healthy fats and flavor.

Preparation Time: 20 minutes

2. Lentil Soup

Ingredients:

> ➤ 1 cup dry lentils, rinsed
> ➤ 4 cups vegetable broth

- ➢ 1 onion, diced
- ➢ 2 carrots, diced
- ➢ 2 celery stalks, diced
- ➢ 2 cloves garlic, minced
- ➢ 1 teaspoon dried thyme
- ➢ 1 teaspoon dried rosemary
- ➢ Salt and pepper to taste
- ➢ Fresh parsley for garnish (optional)

Instructions:

- ➢ In a large pot, sauté onion, carrots, celery, and garlic until softened.
- ➢ Add lentils, vegetable broth, dried thyme, dried rosemary, salt, and pepper to the pot. Bring to a boil.
- ➢ Reduce heat, cover, and simmer for 25-30 minutes, or until lentils are tender.
- ➢ Adjust seasoning if needed and serve hot, garnished with fresh parsley if desired.

Health Benefits:

- ➢ Lentils are rich in protein, fiber, and iron, supporting energy levels and digestive health.

➢ This soup is hydrating and comforting, perfect for seniors with Sjögren's syndrome.

Preparation Time: 40 minutes

3. Mediterranean Hummus Wrap

Ingredients:

➢ Whole grain wrap or lavash

➢ Hummus (store-bought or homemade)

➢ Sliced cucumber

➢ Sliced tomato

➢ Sliced red bell pepper

➢ Kalamata olives, sliced

➢ Fresh spinach leaves

➢ Optional add-ons: sliced red onion, shredded carrots, chopped parsley

Instructions:

➢ Spread a generous layer of hummus onto the center of the wrap or lavash.

➢ Layer cucumber slices, tomato slices, red bell pepper slices, olives, and spinach leaves on top of the hummus.

➤ Add any optional add-ons, if desired.

➤ Roll up the wrap tightly, tucking in the sides as you go.

➤ Slice the wrap in half diagonally and serve immediately or wrap in parchment paper for later.

Health Benefits:

➤ This Mediterranean-inspired wrap is loaded with fiber, vitamins, minerals, and healthy fats from the vegetables, olives, and hummus.

➤ It's a satisfying and flavorful lunch option.

Preparation Time: 10 minutes

4. Roasted Vegetable Quinoa Bowl

Ingredients:

➤ 1 cup cooked quinoa

➤ Assorted roasted vegetables (e.g., sweet potatoes, Brussels sprouts, cauliflower, bell peppers)

➤ Mixed greens (e.g., spinach, kale)

➤ Balsamic vinaigrette dressing (store-bought or homemade)

Instructions:

> ➢ Preheat the oven to 400°F (200°C). Toss assorted vegetables with olive oil, salt, and pepper on a baking sheet.
> ➢ Roast vegetables in the preheated oven for 20-25 minutes, or until tender and caramelized.
> ➢ In a bowl, layer cooked quinoa, roasted vegetables, and mixed greens.
> ➢ Drizzle with balsamic vinaigrette dressing and toss to combine.
> ➢ Serve warm or at room temperature.

Health Benefits:

> ➢ This quinoa bowl is packed with fiber, vitamins, minerals, and antioxidants from the vegetables and quinoa.
> ➢ The balsamic vinaigrette adds flavor without added salt.

Preparation Time: 30 minutes

5. Black Bean and Corn Salad

Ingredients:

- ➢ 1 can black beans, drained and rinsed
- ➢ 1 cup corn kernels (fresh, frozen, or canned)
- ➢ 1 bell pepper, diced
- ➢ 1/4 cup red onion, diced
- ➢ 1/4 cup fresh cilantro, chopped
- ➢ Juice of 1 lime
- ➢ 1 tablespoon olive oil
- ➢ Salt and pepper to taste
- ➢ Avocado slices for garnish (optional)

Instructions:

- ➢ In a large bowl, combine black beans, corn kernels, diced bell pepper, diced red onion, and chopped cilantro.
- ➢ Drizzle with lime juice and olive oil. Season with salt and pepper to taste.
- ➢ Toss to combine all ingredients evenly.
- ➢ Garnish with avocado slices, if desired.
- ➢ Serve chilled or at room temperature.

Health Benefits:

> ➤ This salad is rich in fiber, protein, vitamins, and minerals from the beans, corn, and vegetables. It's refreshing and hydrating, perfect for a light lunch.

Preparation Time: 15 minutes

6. Stuffed Bell Peppers

Ingredients:

> ➤ Bell peppers, halved and seeds removed
> ➤ Cooked quinoa or brown rice
> ➤ Cooked lentils or black beans
> ➤ Sautéed vegetables (e.g., onions, mushrooms, spinach)
> ➤ Tomato sauce or salsa
> ➤ Vegan cheese (optional)
> ➤ Fresh herbs for garnish (e.g., parsley, basil)

Instructions:

> ➤ Preheat the oven to 375°F (190°C). Place halved bell peppers on a baking sheet lined with parchment paper.

- In a large bowl, mix cooked quinoa or brown rice, cooked lentils or black beans, sautéed vegetables, and tomato sauce or salsa.
- Stuff each bell pepper half with the quinoa mixture.
- If using vegan cheese, sprinkle it on top of the stuffed peppers.
- Bake in the preheated oven for 25-30 minutes, or until the peppers are tender.
- Garnish with fresh herbs before serving.

Health Benefits:

- Stuffed bell peppers are a nutritious and satisfying meal option, providing fiber, protein, vitamins, and minerals.
- They're customizable and easy to make ahead for convenient lunches.

Preparation Time: 45 minutes

7. Veggie Stir-Fry with Tofu

Ingredients:

- 1 block extra-firm tofu, pressed and cubed

- Assorted vegetables (e.g., bell peppers, broccoli, carrots, snap peas)
- 2 cloves garlic, minced
- 1 tablespoon ginger, minced
- Soy sauce or tamari
- Sesame oil
- Cooked brown rice or quinoa for serving

Instructions:

- Heat sesame oil in a large skillet or wok over medium-high heat.
- Add cubed tofu to the skillet and cook until golden brown on all sides. Remove tofu from the skillet and set aside.
- In the same skillet, add minced garlic and ginger. Sauté for 1-2 minutes until fragrant.
- Add assorted vegetables to the skillet and stir-fry until tender-crisp.
- Return cooked tofu to the skillet. Drizzle with soy sauce or tamari and toss to coat evenly.
- Serve stir-fried tofu and vegetables over cooked brown rice or quinoa.

Health Benefits:

> This veggie stir-fry is a protein-rich and nutrient-dense meal, providing fiber, vitamins, minerals, and antioxidants from the tofu and vegetables. It's flavorful and satisfying.

Preparation Time: 30 minutes

8. Chickpea Salad Sandwich

Ingredients:

> 1 can chickpeas, drained and rinsed
>
> 1/4 cup diced celery
>
> 1/4 cup diced red onion
>
> 1/4 cup diced pickles
>
> 2 tablespoons vegan mayonnaise
>
> 1 tablespoon Dijon mustard
>
> Salt and pepper to taste
>
> Whole grain bread or wraps
>
> Lettuce leaves and tomato slices for serving

Instructions:

> In a bowl, mash chickpeas with a fork or potato masher until partially mashed.

➢ Add diced celery, red onion, pickles, vegan mayonnaise, Dijon mustard, salt, and pepper to the bowl. Stir to combine all ingredients.

➢ Spread chickpea salad onto whole grain bread or wraps.

➢ Top with lettuce leaves and tomato slices.

➢ Serve sandwiches immediately or wrap in parchment paper for later.

Health Benefits:

➢ This chickpea salad is a delicious and satisfying plant-based alternative to traditional tuna or chicken salad. It's high in fiber, protein, and essential nutrients.

Preparation Time: 15 minutes

9. Veggie and Hummus Wrap

Ingredients:

➢ Whole grain wrap or lavash

➢ Hummus (store-bought or homemade)

➢ Sliced cucumber

➢ Sliced bell peppers

- ➢ Shredded carrots
- ➢ Mixed greens (e.g., spinach, arugula)
- ➢ Optional add-ons: avocado slices, sliced tomatoes, sprouts

Instructions:

- ➢ Spread a layer of hummus onto the center of the wrap or lavash.
- ➢ Layer sliced cucumber, bell peppers, shredded carrots, and mixed greens on top of the hummus.
- ➢ Add any optional add-ons, if desired.
- ➢ Roll up the wrap tightly, tucking in the sides as you go.
- ➢ Slice the wrap in half diagonally and serve immediately or wrap in parchment paper for later.

Health Benefits:

- ➢ This veggie and hummus wrap is loaded with fiber, vitamins, minerals, and healthy fats, providing sustained energy and essential nutrients. It's light, refreshing, and perfect for lunch.

Preparation Time: 10 minutes

10. Vegan Buddha Bowl

Ingredients:

- ➢ Cooked quinoa or brown rice
- ➢ Roasted or steamed vegetables (e.g., sweet potatoes, broccoli, cauliflower, carrots)
- ➢ Massaged kale or spinach
- ➢ Avocado slices
- ➢ Drizzle of tahini or lemon-tahini dressing (see recipe #1)
- ➢ Optional add-ons: cooked lentils or chickpeas, sautéed tofu or tempeh, sliced radishes, pumpkin seeds

Instructions:

- ➢ Arrange cooked quinoa or brown rice, roasted or steamed vegetables, massaged kale or spinach, and avocado slices in a bowl.
- ➢ Add any optional add-ons, if desired.
- ➢ Drizzle with tahini or lemon-tahini dressing.
- ➢ Serve immediately.

Health Benefits:

> This vegan Buddha bowl is a nutrient-packed meal, providing a balance of carbohydrates, protein, healthy fats, fiber, vitamins, and minerals. It's customizable and satisfying.

Preparation Time: 30 minutes

Plant-Based Sjogren Syndrome Diet Dinner Recipes for Seniors

1. Lentil Soup

Ingredients:

> 1 cup dried lentils, rinsed

> 4 cups vegetable broth

> 1 onion, chopped

> 2 carrots, diced

> 2 celery stalks, chopped

> 2 cloves garlic, minced

> 1 teaspoon ground cumin

> 1 teaspoon paprika

> Salt and pepper to taste

> Fresh parsley for garnish (optional)

Instructions:

> ➤ In a large pot, sauté onion, carrots, and celery in a bit of vegetable broth until softened.
> ➤ Add garlic, cumin, and paprika. Cook for another minute.
> ➤ Add lentils and vegetable broth. Bring to a boil, then reduce heat and simmer for 20-25 minutes, until lentils are tender.
> ➤ Season with salt and pepper to taste.
> ➤ Serve hot, garnished with fresh parsley if desired.

Health Benefits:

> ➤ Lentils are rich in protein, fiber, and various vitamins and minerals.
> ➤ This soup is hearty, comforting, and provides essential nutrients for seniors with Sjögren's syndrome.

Preparation Time: 40 minutes

2. Chickpea and Vegetable Stir-Fry

Ingredients:

> ➤ 1 can chickpeas, drained and rinsed

- ➤ 2 cups mixed vegetables (e.g., bell peppers, broccoli, snap peas)
- ➤ 2 cloves garlic, minced
- ➤ 1 tablespoon ginger, minced
- ➤ 2 tablespoons soy sauce or tamari
- ➤ 1 tablespoon maple syrup or honey
- ➤ 1 teaspoon sesame oil
- ➤ Cooked brown rice or quinoa for serving
- ➤ Sesame seeds for garnish (optional)
- ➤ Green onions, sliced (optional)

Instructions:

- ➤ Heat sesame oil in a large skillet over medium heat.
- ➤ Add minced garlic and ginger, and sauté for 1-2 minutes until fragrant.
- ➤ Add mixed vegetables and chickpeas to the skillet, and stir-fry for 5-7 minutes until vegetables are tender-crisp.
- ➤ In a small bowl, whisk together soy sauce and maple syrup. Pour over the vegetables and chickpeas, and toss to coat evenly.

> Serve stir-fry over cooked brown rice or quinoa, garnished with sesame seeds and sliced green onions if desired.

Health Benefits:

> Chickpeas are a good source of plant-based protein and fiber, while vegetables provide vitamins, minerals, and antioxidants.
> This stir-fry is flavorful, satisfying, and easy to digest.

Preparation Time: 20 minutes

3. Stuffed Bell Peppers

Ingredients:

> 4 large bell peppers, halved and seeds removed
> 1 cup cooked quinoa or brown rice
> 1 can black beans, drained and rinsed
> 1 cup corn kernels (fresh, frozen, or canned)
> 1 cup salsa
> 1 teaspoon ground cumin
> 1 teaspoon chili powder
> Salt and pepper to taste

- ➢ Fresh cilantro for garnish (optional)
- ➢ Avocado slices for serving (optional)

Instructions:

- ➢ Preheat oven to 375°F (190°C).
- ➢ In a large bowl, mix together cooked quinoa or brown rice, black beans, corn kernels, salsa, ground cumin, chili powder, salt, and pepper.
- ➢ Stuff each bell pepper half with the quinoa mixture, pressing down gently to fill.
- ➢ Place stuffed bell peppers in a baking dish, cover with foil, and bake for 25-30 minutes until peppers are tender.
- ➢ Remove foil and bake for an additional 5 minutes to lightly brown the tops.
- ➢ Serve stuffed bell peppers hot, garnished with fresh cilantro and avocado slices if desired.

Health Benefits:

- ➢ Bell peppers are rich in vitamin C and antioxidants, while black beans provide protein, fiber, and essential nutrients.

➤ This dish is satisfying, nutrient-dense, and easy to digest.

Preparation Time: 45 minutes

4. Mushroom and Spinach Pasta

Ingredients:

➤ 8 oz (225g) whole wheat or gluten-free pasta

➤ 2 cups sliced mushrooms

➤ 2 cups fresh spinach

➤ 2 cloves garlic, minced

➤ 1/4 cup vegetable broth or white wine

➤ 2 tablespoons nutritional yeast (optional)

➤ Salt and pepper to taste

➤ Fresh parsley for garnish (optional)

➤ Vegan parmesan cheese for serving (optional)

Instructions:

➤ Cook pasta according to package instructions until al dente. Drain and set aside.

➤ In a large skillet, sauté sliced mushrooms and minced garlic in vegetable broth or white wine until mushrooms are softened.

- ➢ Add fresh spinach to the skillet and cook until wilted.

- ➢ Stir in cooked pasta and nutritional yeast (if using). Season with salt and pepper to taste.

- ➢ Cook for an additional 2-3 minutes until heated through.

- ➢ Serve hot, garnished with fresh parsley and vegan parmesan cheese if desired.

Health Benefits:

- ➢ Whole wheat pasta provides fiber and complex carbohydrates, while mushrooms and spinach offer vitamins, minerals, and antioxidants.

- ➢ This pasta dish is filling, flavorful, and nutritious.

Preparation Time: 20 minutes

5. Tofu and Vegetable Stir-Fry

Ingredients:

- ➢ 1 block firm tofu, pressed and cubed

- ➢ 2 cups mixed vegetables (e.g., bell peppers, broccoli, carrots)

- ➢ 2 cloves garlic, minced

- ➢ 1 tablespoon ginger, minced

- ➢ 2 tablespoons soy sauce or tamari
- ➢ 1 tablespoon maple syrup or honey
- ➢ 1 teaspoon sesame oil
- ➢ Cooked brown rice or quinoa for serving
- ➢ Sesame seeds for garnish (optional)
- ➢ Green onions, sliced (optional)

Instructions:

- ➢ Heat sesame oil in a large skillet over medium heat.
- ➢ Add cubed tofu to the skillet and cook until golden brown on all sides, about 5-7 minutes. Remove tofu from skillet and set aside.
- ➢ In the same skillet, add minced garlic and ginger, and sauté for 1-2 minutes until fragrant.
- ➢ Add mixed vegetables to the skillet and stir-fry for 5-7 minutes until tender-crisp.
- ➢ Return cooked tofu to the skillet, and add soy sauce and maple syrup. Toss to coat evenly.
- ➢ Serve stir-fry over cooked brown rice or quinoa, garnished with sesame seeds and sliced green onions if desired.

Health Benefits:

> ➤ Tofu is a versatile source of plant-based protein, while mixed vegetables provide vitamins, minerals, and fiber. This stir-fry is flavorful, satisfying, and easy to digest.

Preparation Time: 30 minutes

6. Quinoa Salad with Roasted Vegetables

Ingredients:

> ➤ 1 cup cooked quinoa
> ➤ 2 cups mixed roasted vegetables (e.g., bell peppers, zucchini, eggplant)
> ➤ 1/4 cup cherry tomatoes, halved
> ➤ Handful of baby spinach
> ➤ 2 tablespoons balsamic vinegar
> ➤ 1 tablespoon olive oil
> ➤ Salt and pepper to taste
> ➤ Fresh basil for garnish (optional)
> ➤ Vegan feta cheese for serving (optional)

Instructions:

> In a large bowl, combine cooked quinoa, roasted vegetables, cherry tomatoes, and baby spinach.
> In a small bowl, whisk together balsamic vinegar, olive oil, salt, and pepper.
> Pour dressing over the quinoa salad and toss to coat evenly.
> Serve salad garnished with fresh basil and vegan feta cheese if desired.

Health Benefits:

> Quinoa is a complete protein and a good source of fiber and minerals, while roasted vegetables offer vitamins, antioxidants, and fiber.
> This salad is light, refreshing, and nutrient-dense.

Preparation Time: 30 minutes

7. Vegan Lentil Shepherd's Pie

Ingredients:

> 2 cups cooked lentils
> 1 onion, chopped
> 2 carrots, diced

- 2 celery stalks, chopped
- 2 cloves garlic, minced
- 1 cup frozen peas
- 1 cup vegetable broth
- 2 tablespoons tomato paste
- 1 teaspoon dried thyme
- Salt and pepper to taste
- Mashed potatoes (prepared separately)
- Fresh parsley for garnish (optional)

Instructions:

- Preheat oven to 375°F (190°C).
- In a large skillet, sauté onion, carrots, celery, and garlic until softened.
- Add cooked lentils, frozen peas, vegetable broth, tomato paste, dried thyme, salt, and pepper to the skillet. Stir to combine.
- Cook for 5-7 minutes until heated through and flavors are blended.
- Transfer lentil mixture to a baking dish and spread evenly.
- Top with mashed potatoes, spreading to cover the lentil mixture.

- ➤ Bake in the preheated oven for 25-30 minutes until bubbly and lightly golden.
- ➤ Serve hot, garnished with fresh parsley if desired.

Health Benefits:

- ➤ Lentils are rich in protein, fiber, and various vitamins and minerals, making them an excellent plant-based protein source. This shepherd's pie is hearty, comforting, and nutrient-dense.

Preparation Time: 45 minutes

8. Mediterranean Quinoa Salad

Ingredients:

- ➤ 1 cup cooked quinoa
- ➤ 1 cup cherry tomatoes, halved
- ➤ 1 cucumber, diced
- ➤ 1/4 cup sliced Kalamata olives
- ➤ 1/4 cup diced red onion
- ➤ 2 tablespoons chopped fresh parsley
- ➤ 2 tablespoons extra virgin olive oil
- ➤ 1 tablespoon lemon juice
- ➤ 1 teaspoon dried oregano

- ➢ Salt and pepper to taste
- ➢ Vegan feta cheese for serving (optional)

Instructions:

- ➢ In a large bowl, combine cooked quinoa, cherry tomatoes, cucumber, Kalamata olives, red onion, and chopped parsley.
- ➢ In a small bowl, whisk together extra virgin olive oil, lemon juice, dried oregano, salt, and pepper.
- ➢ Pour dressing over the quinoa salad and toss to coat evenly.
- ➢ Serve salad topped with vegan feta cheese if desired.

Health Benefits:

- ➢ Quinoa is a complete protein and a good source of fiber and minerals, while vegetables and olives provide vitamins, antioxidants, and healthy fats. This salad is light, refreshing, and packed with flavor.

Preparation Time: 20 minutes

9. Vegetable Curry with Coconut Milk

Ingredients:

- 2 cups mixed vegetables (e.g., cauliflower, carrots, bell peppers, peas)
- 1 onion, chopped
- 2 cloves garlic, minced
- 1 tablespoon grated ginger
- 1 can (14 oz) coconut milk
- 2 tablespoons curry powder
- 1 tablespoon tomato paste
- 1 tablespoon maple syrup or honey
- Salt and pepper to taste
- Fresh cilantro for garnish (optional)
- Cooked brown rice or quinoa for serving

Instructions:

- In a large skillet, sauté chopped onion, minced garlic, and grated ginger until softened.
- Add mixed vegetables to the skillet and cook for 5-7 minutes until slightly tender.
- Stir in curry powder, tomato paste, maple syrup, salt, and pepper.

➢ Pour in coconut milk and bring to a simmer. Cook for 10-15 minutes until vegetables are cooked through and sauce is thickened.

➢ Serve vegetable curry hot, garnished with fresh cilantro, over cooked brown rice or quinoa.

Health Benefits:

➢ Coconut milk adds creaminess and healthy fats to the dish, while vegetables provide vitamins, minerals, and fiber.

➢ This curry is flavorful, comforting, and nutritious.

Preparation Time: 30 minutes

10. Eggplant and Chickpea Tagine

Ingredients:

➢ 1 eggplant, cubed

➢ 1 can chickpeas, drained and rinsed

➢ 1 onion, chopped

➢ 2 cloves garlic, minced

➢ 1 tablespoon grated ginger

➢ 1 can (14 oz) diced tomatoes

➢ 1/4 cup dried apricots, chopped

- ➢ 1 teaspoon ground cumin
- ➢ 1 teaspoon ground coriander
- ➢ 1/2 teaspoon cinnamon
- ➢ Salt and pepper to taste
- ➢ Fresh cilantro for garnish (optional)
- ➢ Cooked couscous or quinoa for serving

Instructions:

- ➢ In a large pot or tagine, sauté chopped onion, minced garlic, and grated ginger until softened.
- ➢ Add cubed eggplant to the pot and cook for 5 minutes until slightly browned.
- ➢ Stir in diced tomatoes, chickpeas, chopped dried apricots, ground cumin, ground coriander, cinnamon, salt, and pepper.
- ➢ Cover and simmer for 20-25 minutes until eggplant is tender and flavors are blended.
- ➢ Serve tagine hot, garnished with fresh cilantro, over cooked couscous or quinoa.

Health Benefits:

- ➢ Eggplant and chickpeas are rich in fiber and antioxidants, while dried apricots add natural sweetness and vitamins. This tagine is aromatic, satisfying, and packed with nutrients.

Preparation Time: 40 minutes

Plant-Based Sjogren Syndrome Diet Snacks Recipes for Seniors

1. Hummus with Veggie Sticks

Ingredients:

- 1 cup cooked chickpeas (canned or cooked from dried)
- 2 tablespoons tahini
- 2 tablespoons lemon juice
- 1 garlic clove, minced
- 1/4 teaspoon cumin
- Salt and pepper to taste
- Assorted vegetable sticks (carrots, cucumbers, bell peppers)

Instructions:

- In a food processor, combine chickpeas, tahini, lemon juice, minced garlic, cumin, salt, and pepper.

> Blend until smooth, adding a splash of water if needed to reach desired consistency.

> Serve hummus with assorted vegetable sticks for dipping.

Health Benefits:

> Hummus is rich in plant-based protein and fiber from chickpeas, while vegetables provide vitamins, minerals, and antioxidants.

> This snack supports hydration and digestive health.

Preparation Time: 10 minutes

2. Trail Mix

Ingredients:

> 1/2 cup raw almonds

> 1/2 cup raw cashews

> 1/4 cup pumpkin seeds

> 1/4 cup dried cranberries

> 1/4 cup dried apricots, chopped

Instructions:

> In a bowl, combine almonds, cashews, pumpkin seeds, dried cranberries, and chopped apricots.

- ➢ Mix well to combine.
- ➢ Store trail mix in an airtight container for snacking on-the-go.

Health Benefits:

- ➢ Trail mix provides a combination of protein, healthy fats, and carbohydrates, offering sustained energy and essential nutrients.
- ➢ Nuts and seeds are rich in vitamins, minerals, and antioxidants.

Preparation Time: 5 minutes

3. Rice Cake with Almond Butter and Banana

Ingredients:

- ➢ 1 rice cake
- ➢ 1 tablespoon almond butter
- ➢ 1/2 banana, sliced
- ➢ Drizzle of honey or maple syrup (optional)

Instructions:

- ➢ Spread almond butter evenly onto the rice cake.
- ➢ Top with sliced banana.
- ➢ Drizzle with honey or maple syrup, if desired.

➢ Serve immediately.

Health Benefits:

➢ Rice cakes provide a crunchy base, while almond butter offers healthy fats and protein. Bananas add natural sweetness, fiber, and potassium.

Preparation Time: 5 minutes

4. Energy Bites

Ingredients:

➢ 1 cup rolled oats
➢ 1/2 cup almond butter
➢ 1/4 cup maple syrup or honey
➢ 1/4 cup shredded coconut
➢ 1/4 cup mini chocolate chips or dried fruit (optional)
➢ 1 teaspoon vanilla extract
➢ Pinch of salt

Instructions:

➢ In a bowl, mix together rolled oats, almond butter, maple syrup or honey, shredded coconut, chocolate chips or dried fruit (if using), vanilla extract, and a pinch of salt.

- ➤ Roll the mixture into small balls using your hands.
- ➤ Place energy bites on a baking sheet lined with parchment paper.
- ➤ Chill in the refrigerator for at least 30 minutes before serving.

Health Benefits:

- ➤ Energy bites are a convenient and portable snack rich in fiber, protein, and healthy fats.
- ➤ They provide a quick source of energy and satisfy hunger between meals.

Preparation Time: 15 minutes (plus chilling time)

5. Veggie Nori Rolls

Ingredients:

- ➤ Nori sheets
- ➤ Cooked quinoa or brown rice
- ➤ Sliced avocado
- ➤ Sliced cucumber
- ➤ Shredded carrots
- ➤ Sliced bell peppers
- ➤ Tahini or hummus for dipping

Instructions:

> ➢ Place a nori sheet on a flat surface.
> ➢ Spread a thin layer of cooked quinoa or brown rice over the nori sheet.
> ➢ Arrange sliced avocado, cucumber, shredded carrots, and bell peppers along the bottom edge of the nori sheet.
> ➢ Roll the nori sheet tightly into a cylinder, using a bit of water to seal the edge.
> ➢ Slice the roll into bite-sized pieces using a sharp knife.
> ➢ Serve with tahini or hummus for dipping.

Health Benefits:

> ➢ Nori rolls are a nutritious and flavorful snack packed with vitamins, minerals, and fiber from vegetables and whole grains.
> ➢ They provide a satisfying crunch and arc low in calories.

Preparation Time: 20 minutes

6. Apple Slices with Nut Butter

Ingredients:

- ➢ 1 apple, sliced
- ➢ 2 tablespoons almond butter or peanut butter
- ➢ Cinnamon (optional)

Instructions:

- ➢ Slice the apple into thin wedges.
- ➢ Spread almond butter or peanut butter on each apple slice.
- ➢ Sprinkle with cinnamon, if desired.
- ➢ Serve immediately.

Health Benefits:

- ➢ Apples are rich in fiber, vitamins, and antioxidants, while nut butter provides protein, healthy fats, and essential nutrients. This snack is satisfying and provides sustained energy.

Preparation Time: 5 minutes

7. Greek Yogurt with Berries

Ingredients:

- 1/2 cup dairy-free Greek yogurt (e.g., almond or coconut yogurt)
- Mixed berries (e.g., strawberries, blueberries, raspberries)
- Drizzle of honey or maple syrup (optional)

Instructions:

- Spoon Greek yogurt into a bowl.
- Top with mixed berries.
- Drizzle with honey or maple syrup, if desired.
- Serve chilled.

Health Benefits:

- Greek yogurt is high in protein and probiotics, which support gut health and immune function. Berries add antioxidants, vitamins, and fiber.

Preparation Time: 5 minutes

8. Edamame

Ingredients:

- ➢ Frozen edamame pods
- ➢ Sea salt

Instructions:

- ➢ Cook edamame pods according to package instructions (usually boiling or steaming for a few minutes).
- ➢ Drain and rinse the cooked edamame pods.
- ➢ Sprinkle with sea salt.
- ➢ Serve warm or chilled.

Health Benefits:

- ➢ Edamame is a soybean rich in protein, fiber, vitamins, and minerals. It's a convenient and nutritious snack that helps promote fullness and satiety.

Preparation Time: 10 minutes

9. Veggie Stuffed Mini Peppers

Ingredients:

- Mini bell peppers, halved and deseeded
- Hummus or guacamole
- Cherry tomatoes, halved
- Cucumber slices
- Fresh basil leaves
- Balsamic glaze (optional)

Instructions:

- Fill each mini pepper half with hummus or guacamole.
- Top with cherry tomato halves, cucumber slices, and fresh basil leaves.
- Drizzle with balsamic glaze, if desired.
- Serve immediately.

Health Benefits:

- Mini peppers are low in calories and rich in vitamins, while hummus or guacamole provides healthy fats, protein, and fiber. This snack is colorful, crunchy, and satisfying.

Preparation Time: 10 minutes

10. Baked Sweet Potato Fries

Ingredients:

- 2 medium sweet potatoes, peeled and cut into fries
- 1 tablespoon olive oil
- 1 teaspoon paprika
- 1/2 teaspoon garlic powder
- Salt and pepper to taste

Instructions:

- Preheat the oven to 425°F (220°C) and line a baking sheet with parchment paper.
- In a bowl, toss sweet potato fries with olive oil, paprika, garlic powder, salt, and pepper until evenly coated.
- Arrange sweet potato fries in a single layer on the prepared baking sheet.
- Bake for 20-25 minutes, flipping halfway through, until fries are golden brown and crispy.
- Remove from the oven and let cool slightly before serving.

Health Benefits:

> ➤ Sweet potatoes are rich in vitamins, minerals, and antioxidants, while olive oil provides heart-healthy fats. Baked sweet potato fries are a nutritious alternative to traditional fries.

Preparation Time: 30 minutes

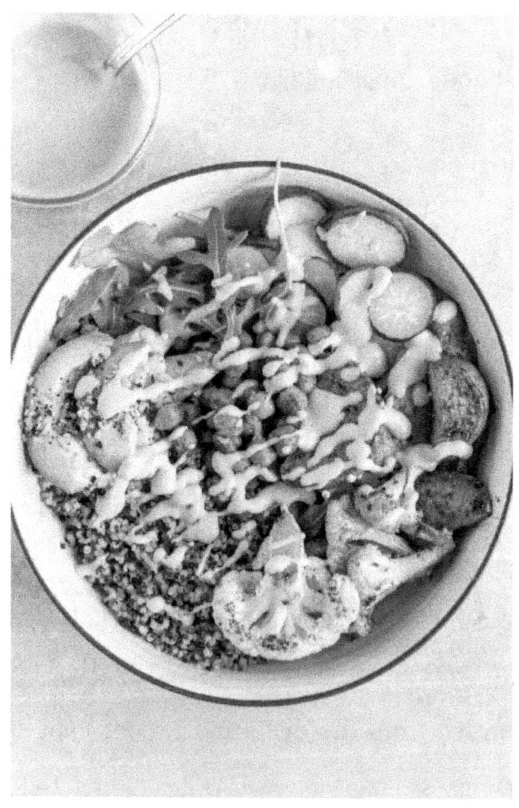

CONCLUSION

Adopting a plant-based diet tailored for seniors with Sjögren's syndrome offers a wealth of benefits for both their physical health and overall well-being.

By emphasizing whole, minimally processed plant foods rich in nutrients, antioxidants, and anti-inflammatory compounds, seniors can effectively manage symptoms associated with Sjögren's syndrome while supporting their immune system and promoting optimal health.

From hydrating chia seed puddings to nourishing veggie-packed meals like tofu scrambles and sweet potato hash, the diverse array of plant-based recipes provides seniors with delicious and nutritious options for every meal and snack.

These recipes not only address the specific dietary needs of seniors with Sjögren's syndrome but also cater to their taste preferences and dietary restrictions, ensuring a sustainable and enjoyable eating experience.

Furthermore, the principles of a plant-based diet empower seniors to take control of their health by making informed dietary choices that align with their individual needs and goals.

By working closely with healthcare providers or registered dietitians to develop personalized meal plans, seniors can embark on a journey towards improved vitality, enhanced symptom management, and a greater quality of life.

Incorporating plant-based eating into the daily routine of seniors with Sjögren's syndrome not only nourishes the body but also nourishes the spirit, fostering a sense of empowerment, resilience, and well-being.

With each nutritious bite, seniors can take a step closer to thriving in their golden years, enjoying a life of vitality and fulfillment.

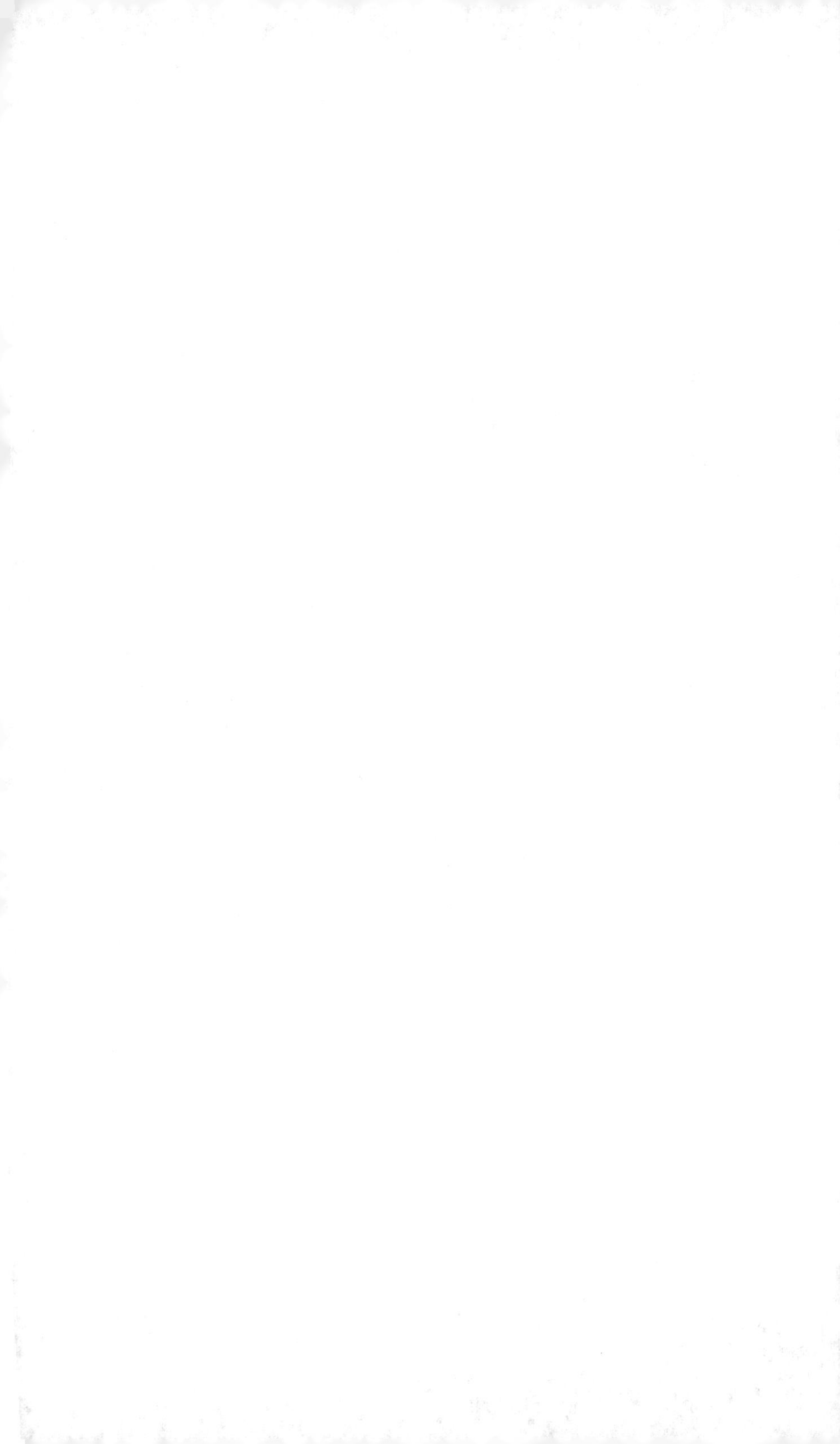